FEED

YOUR POTENTIAL

HOW TO FUEL YOUR SOUL

AND TAKE CONTROL!

DORRON BLUMBERG

ISBN-13: 978-1500966294

Printed in the United States of America Published by Dorron Blumberg
Visit www.dorronblumberg.com Publisher's Note:
This book is written for educational purposes only and is not intended for the use of any type of psychotherapy or treatment.

Blumberg, Dorron
Feed Your Potential: How To Fuel Your Soul and Take Control

1. Sport Psychology
2. Sports Performance
3. Fitness and Health
4. Nutrition Education

This book is dedicated to you!

Get ready to feed your potential by developing key areas of your life. Results occur when you take the first step in the direction of your goals.

Stay the course, be yourself, and always be open to becoming a better version of you. Be proud of your accomplishments, treat yourself and others with love, and do your best.

The best time to take action is now!

Contents

About Dorron

Dorron Blumberg is originally from Johannesburg, South Africa. He has grown up as an athlete his entire life living in South Africa, Texas, and South Florida. As a young man, he swam and ranked nationally as a youth athlete. After competing as a swimmer, he went on to play football in high school, making the All-County team, the Broward All-Star team, and receiving a scholarship for a strong character on and off the field. After high-school, he went on to play football for Florida Atlantic University (FAU) on their first inaugural team.

His sporting career and life led him to pursue his bachelor's degree from Florida Atlantic University in Exercise Science and Health Promotion. He then went on to receive his Master's Degree in Sport & Performance Psychology from The University of the Rockies.

In addition to the degrees completed, Dorron has the following certifications:

- Fitness Institute International - Certified Personal Training Specialist (CPTS)
- National Strength and Conditioning Association - Certified Personal Trainer (CPT) and a Certified Strength and Conditioning Specialist (CSCS)
- Life Success Consultant,
- Performance Edge Coach
- Level 1 & 2 Training for Warriors Coach
- AED/CPR/First Aid

Dorron has over 20 years' experience in the industry and competed in several races, triathlons, and is an ultimate athlete champion.

He currently works with fitness enthusiasts, coaches, athletes, and professional business men/women.

I am the proud son of a father who has never given up on his dreams. He always inspires me to work hard and do my best. I have two amazing brothers, three sweet dogs, a beautiful fiancee, and a fantastic mother.

Introduction

Feed Your Potential will empower you to fuel your soul and take control! Feed Your Potential will get your mind and body ready for performing at your best. Throughout this book, there will be exercises to complete. Take your time to complete and apply them to your life.

I have personally applied these exercises to my own life and clients I have worked with. They have all improved in their life and sport. I strongly believe the information in this book will do the same for you.

I highly recommend that you keep a journal beside you and take notes along with completing the exercises. Write down any ideas that manifest in your mind and use them if they align with your purpose. Use this book as a resource for improving your sport, business, and life.

One of my hobbies is playing the guitar, and it takes me hundreds of repetitions to learn songs and get the right sounds down. I encourage you to write down your goals and repeat them often.

We all have a journey and purpose in life. Keep positively minded people around you and be grateful along your journey.

Feed Your Potential is broken down into different chapters. The book begins with a self-assessment. Then you will define your purpose, vision, and goals. You will learn different mind training tools and the power behind a performance journal. Other chapters involve mind muscles, emotional intelligence, peak performance, nutrition, fitness, leadership, and growth.

Feed Your Potential is your guide for feeding your mind, business, nutritional, and physical game. Enjoy the material inside this book and take action on your goals.

I have been a student of fitness, health, and nutrition. Before doing any physical activities or applying the nutritional advice in this book, please consult with your doctor if needed. Get all your vitals checked and ensure you are in proper health.

In order to Feed Your Potential, you will need:

1. **Courage:** Mental toughness to overcome distractions, temptations, and negative minded individuals that will try and deter you from your goals!
2. **Strength:** Power to keep yourself motivated, stick to goals, and fortitude to win!
3. **Vitality:** Consistency with your supplementation and eating habits.

Making a choice to improve your lifestyle and nutrition begins with the right mind-set. The way you think creates your habits, and those habits create actions. Your actions create the results you are getting in life. If you are not happy with the results, then you need to change the way you think.

Apply these instant tips to start feeding your potential.

Start your day with 5-10 minutes away from technology. Spend this time breathing, drinking water, and visualizing your goals.

Be kinder to people in your life. Listen more, judge less, and ask more Questions.

Spend more time on personal growth and development. Invest in audio books or video, attend educational seminars. Read, listen to audio books and podcasts.

Take care of your stress. Exercise smartly, spend more time decompressing (stretching, yoga, meditation, etc.), limit toxic foods (processed, fast-foods) and sugary/alcoholic drinks.

Put energy into your passion and others. Follow your heart's desire and give back. Enjoy getting involved with your favorite hobby, growing your career, and volunteering more in your community.

Surround yourself with impact individuals. Spend more time with individuals that will encourage you to grow and support your dreams. Stay positive and bring value to their life as well.

Smile More. Smiling elevates your mood and creates positive energy in your environment. A pleasing personality is always a good thing.

Mind training. Use visualization to prepare yourself to reach optimal conditioning or readiness for your next competition.

Physical training. Make sure you train specifically in the direction of the results you seek. Training the body is a composite of weights, functional movements, body weight, cardiovascular training, stretching, and rest.

Do not over train. Make sure to rest your body and mind. Take some time off. Too much is not a good thing and will lead to burnout. Make sure to give your body rest; you might need to slow down or taper off.

Fuel your body before, during, and after exercise. Proper training requires having glucose in the bloodstream before, during and after exercise. After a workout, refuel your body with a whole meal or a quality protein shake.

Supplement with natural sources! The supplement world is a Multi-billion dollar industry, infused with lots of preservatives, and artificial flavors. Make sure to ask the following questions when choosing to buy supplements:

1. How long has the company been around?
2. Has the supplement been approved by the NSA (National Science Foundation)?
3. Is there medical research on the product, especially from sources other than the company that developed the product?
4. What are the long-term effects?

Assessment

Let's take a look at different parts of your life. Assessing yourself is an important aspect of learning more about you. It is always a good idea to look at your personal life, education, and performance. Rate yourself below on a scale of 1 to 10 (10 being high). Circle your answer and check off each box as you answer the question.

☐ 1. Rate your hygiene habits (i.e., flossing, cleaning your space around you, keeping clothes clean - laundry, etc.)

```
  0   1   2   3   4   5   6   7   8   9   10
```

☐ 2. Rate your ability to handle anxiety/stress (i.e., body language, thoughts, feelings, actions, etc.)

```
  0   1   2   3   4   5   6   7   8   9   10
```

☐ 3. Rate your mental training habits (i.e., journaling, meditation, visualization, etc.)

```
  0   1   2   3   4   5   6   7   8   9   10
```

☐ 4. Rate your drinking/eating habits (i.e., water intake, vegetable consumption, organic protein, high fiber carbs, etc.)

```
  0   1   2   3   4   5   6   7   8   9   10
```

☐ 5. Rate your weight/functional training habits (i.e., resistance exercise in the form of free weight, balls, bands, suspension bands, etc.)

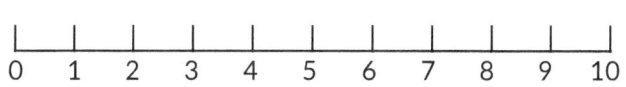

```
  0   1   2   3   4   5   6   7   8   9   10
```

☐ 6. Rate your stretching/core habits (i.e., pilates, yoga, stretching class, etc.)

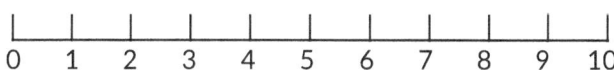

```
  0   1   2   3   4   5   6   7   8   9   10
```

☐ 7. Rae your learning habits (i.e., personal development, podcasts, books, online programs, seminars, etc.)

```
|  |  |  |  |  |  |  |  |  |  |  |
0  1  2  3  4  5  6  7  8  9  10
```

☐ 8. Rate your goal setting habits (i.e., daily goal writing, journaling performance, to do list, etc.)

```
|  |  |  |  |  |  |  |  |  |  |  |
0  1  2  3  4  5  6  7  8  9  10
```

☐ 9. Rate your career happiness (i.e., job enjoyment, purpose, people you work with, etc.)

```
|  |  |  |  |  |  |  |  |  |  |  |
0  1  2  3  4  5  6  7  8  9  10
```

☐ 10. Rate your relationships with loved ones (i.e., how you treat family and friends, communication, support, etc.)

```
|  |  |  |  |  |  |  |  |  |  |  |
0  1  2  3  4  5  6  7  8  9  10
```

☐ 11. Rate your overall attitude (i.e., happy mood, energized, excited, pumped, etc.)

```
|  |  |  |  |  |  |  |  |  |  |  |
0  1  2  3  4  5  6  7  8  9  10
```

☐ 12. Rate your ability to get things done (i.e., complete tasks/assignments/projects, etc.)

```
|  |  |  |  |  |  |  |  |  |  |  |
0  1  2  3  4  5  6  7  8  9  10
```

☐ 13. Rate your financial goals (i.e., own a house, paid the off debt, new car, savings, retirement, etc.)

```
|  |  |  |  |  |  |  |  |  |  |  |
0  1  2  3  4  5  6  7  8  9  10
```

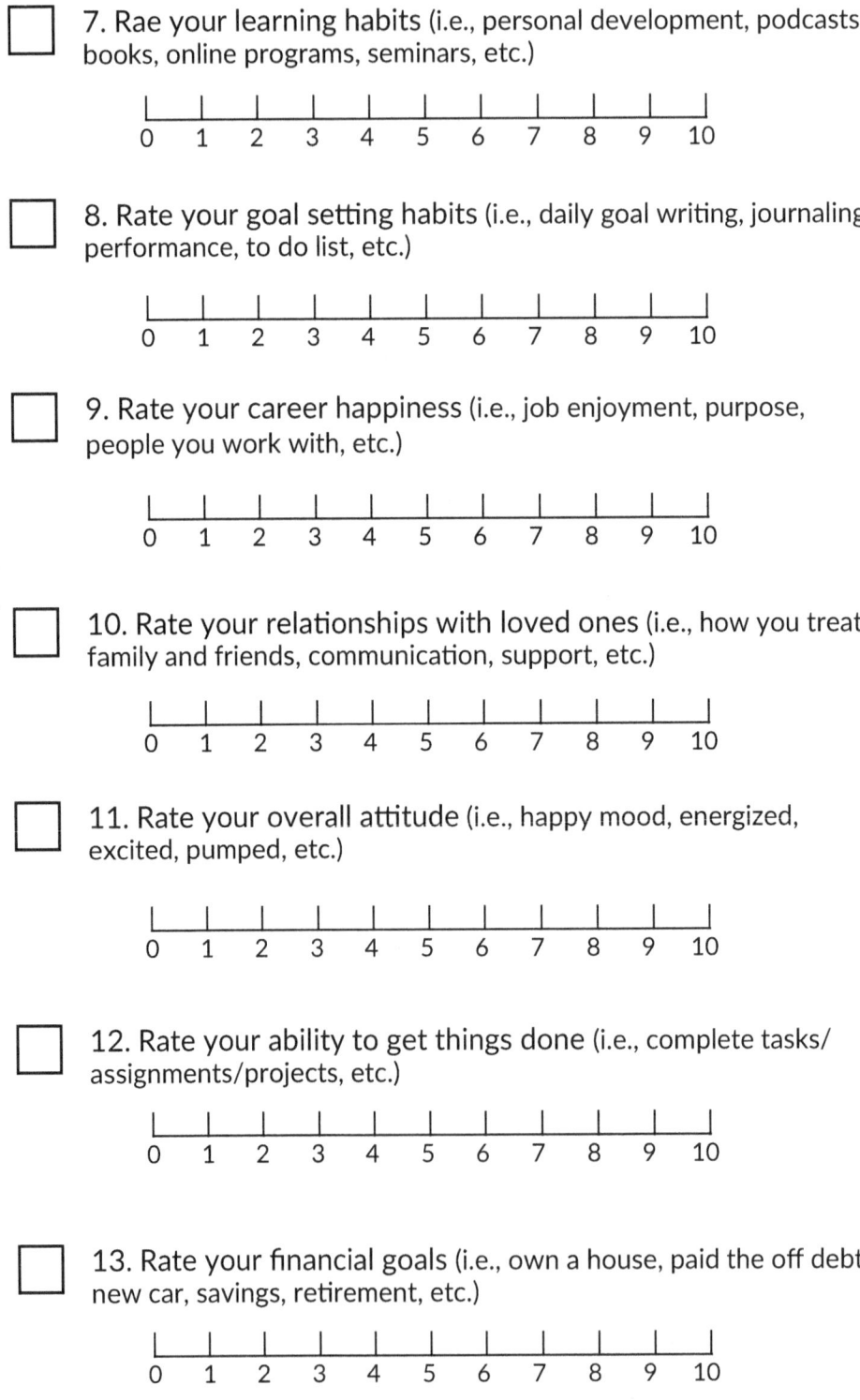

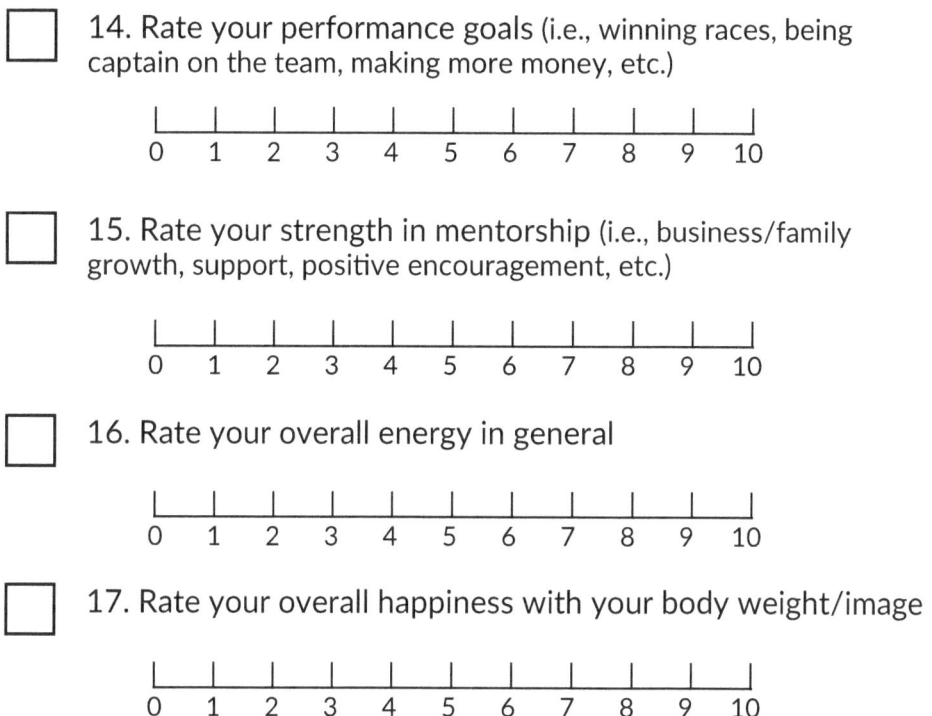

☐ 14. Rate your performance goals (i.e., winning races, being captain on the team, making more money, etc.)

0 1 2 3 4 5 6 7 8 9 10

☐ 15. Rate your strength in mentorship (i.e., business/family growth, support, positive encouragement, etc.)

0 1 2 3 4 5 6 7 8 9 10

☐ 16. Rate your overall energy in general

0 1 2 3 4 5 6 7 8 9 10

☐ 17. Rate your overall happiness with your body weight/image

0 1 2 3 4 5 6 7 8 9 10

Results

_____ TOTAL SCORE x 17 = Answer

Divide Answer by 170 = Score _____

Rank yourself as follows ....

Below 40% ....Weak (need help)
50% to 80%.....Average (doing OK, but could do better)
90% or 100%...Strong (getting good results)

Answer the following questions (Can complete quarterly to yearly)

What is your main goal? (e.g., Build Better Habits, Lose Weight, etc.)

```



```

Who can you lean on for support? (e.g., Family, Friends, Coaches, etc.)

```



```

What thoughts do you need to change or overcome?
(e.g., Negative Self Talk, Close Mind, etc.)

```



```

What obstacles are in your way?
(i.e., Negative Influence, Poor Habits, Stress, etc.)

```



```

HIT and Do your LAPS

Let's take a look at a couple of acronyms I have designed. The first is **HIT**.

I refer to this as:

- Harmonious thoughts
- Impact mind-set
- Target words (self-talk)

This is a great affirmation to use to get you in the right mind-set. Maybe you are feeling tired for your workout or not into your work on a particular day. It is important to hit the switch and turn your thinking around as fast as possible from negative to positive.

"Your thoughts harmonize and impact your mind-set, which in turn generate the actions or words that come out of your mouth."

Here is an example of a negative experience. You are thinking about how you did not get enough sleep the night before, and this impacts your mind. As a result, you begin to tell people you are weak and not looking forward to the day. Your mind is attracting negativity, and your body action reveals sluggishness, laziness, and lack of interest.

Here is an example of a positive experience. You are thinking about how awesome the weather is today. Your mind is impacted and is generating positive vibrations. As a result, you begin to tell people how beautiful the day is and how you feel full of energy. Your mind is attracting positivity, and your body action reveals energy, great posture, and enthusiasm.

My advice: Do your best to attract positive energy. Are you having a bad day? Why not just change it to having bad minutes or moments and do your LAPS.

LAPS work like this:

1. **Lose the Laziness** (e.g., Get tasks completed)

2. **Adjust your Attitude** (Be more positive, sportsmanship)

3. **Practice Skills** (e.g., Sports, Arts, Communication, etc.)

4. **Start Fresh** (Forget about things holding you back. Charge forward with a positive mind-set)

LAPS reminds you to get on your A game. When you HIT the ground running with the right mind-set and do your LAPS daily; you are living a life filled with passion and purpose.

Get ready to define your purpose in the next section.

Your purpose takes education, discipline, and patience to develop. I recommend that you find a quiet place, or discover what works best for you to think.

Golden Circle

"Keep your dreams alive. Understand to achieve anything requires faith and belief in yourself, vision, hard work, determination, and dedication. Remember all things are possible for those who believe.
--Gail Devers

Once you understand why you are doing the things you do, it becomes important to discover what you need to do or what you see in your future. Take a look at these three circles shown below.
This is called the Golden Circle. I learned this from The golden circle by Simon Sinek.

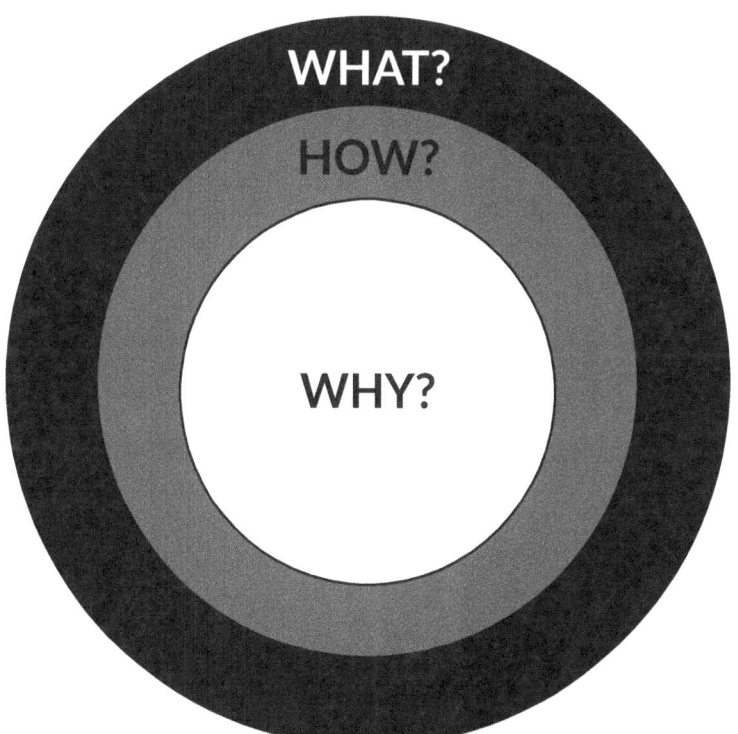

The importance of understanding this Golden Circle is to operate from an inside-out philosophy. The center circle represents your WHY. The next circle is your HOW. The outside circle is your WHAT. The WHY represents your purpose, the HOW represents your goals and your WHAT represents your vision.

As Simon explains, most people know what they do and how to do it. For example, he uses an example of Apple. Say Apple sells you by saying, "we make great computers that are beautifully designed and easy to use." Versus "we challenge the status quo. We make beautifully designed products that are easy to use; we just happen to make good computers want to buy one?"

Sounds much more appealing, right?

You see, the golden circle can be compared to the human brain. The Homo sapiens brain (neocortix) makes up the what section. This part of the brain is responsible for all rational and analytical thought and language. The middle two sections make up the limbic brain. This correlates to all our feelings, human behavior, and decision making.

Thus, influential companies and people start from the inside in to capture their audience. Understand your why and write down the things that make you different.

Write out your why below.

Move Theory

MOVE stands for *motivation, order, vitality, and efficiency*. I believe it is important to know where the **motivation** is coming from. This can come from your health, best performance, family (internal motivation), championship, an award (external motivation).

Order represents a schedule you have in place to help you stay motivated. Also, your cleanliness, and priorities in life. (e.g., developing a to-do list).

Vitality represents your nutrition, hydration, environment, balance, and recovery. Focus on quality over quantity.

Efficiency relates to being able to operate effectively. Are you getting the job done or procrastinating?

Whatever the case is remember to make sure you manage your time and have the energy to get it done right.

Feed Your Potential will inspire you to **MOVE** in the right direction!

Create Your Vision Image

One of the great things you can do is develop a vision image. There are no rules for this exercise. It can be as simple as an image of what you want to look like. It can be an image of your team/company logo that you place on the screen of your tablet, smart phone, or computer screen. It can consist of your performance goals, purpose statement, health, favorite athlete or sport, quote, people in your life, a competition you excelled at in the past or even other goals you have. You can even place images on social media and share your vision with others.

Develop your vision image and place in an area where you can see it daily.

"Find that something to hold onto and drive you to achieve greatness."

Drafting Your Purpose

"There is one quality which one must possess to win, and that is definiteness of purpose, the knowledge of what one wants, and a burning desire to possess it." --Napoleon Hill

Your purpose equates to your why. Your why reflects on your values in life. I like to break down the development of your purpose into five key areas as described below:

1. **Traits:** Positive and negative aspects you need to develop.
2. **Goals:** Personal, education, and performance goals you have for yourself.
3. **Sacrifices:** What are you willing to sacrifice to accomplish your goals.
4. **Hobbies:** What hobbies do you have that compliment your passions in life?
5. **Family/Community:** How can you be closer with your loved ones and community?

It is important to write your goals because it provides a written contract to yourself. Remember that the pen never forgets, but the mind does.

Traits: Write down the two best qualities you have.

Write down two qualities you need to work on.

Goals: Write down your goals for each key area of your life (personal, education, and performance). It is also important to make sure your goals have a time table. I recommend writing out goals for your purpose statement every 90 days.

```



```

Sacrifices: Write down three aspects of your life; you are willing to give up to accomplish your goals.

```



```

Hobbies: Write down three hobbies you have and explain why.

```



```

Family/Community: Write down how you can you be closer with your loved ones and community?

```



```

*Later in this book, I will go into more detail with using a goal setting ladder.

Purpose on a Daily Basis

A good exercise is to ask yourself the following questions every morning when you wake up to empower your purpose:

- What are my main goals today?
- Why do I want accomplish these goals?
- How can I get them done and at what time?
- What resources will I need to assist me?
- Who can support me with my goals?

Challenge your mind to think and write down goals and actions on a regular basis. Follow through with your tasks, exceed people's expectations, go out of your way to get something done, make people feel good, give compliments, befriend people, and follow your heart.

Do what you love best. Make life fun and enjoy putting all the work in on a daily basis.

Find something that you absolutely want to hold onto. It does not matter what life stage you are in; there is always something more that can get you moving. You are different from everyone else, so take the time to discover your true purpose.

Visualization

I believe that visualization is one of the most powerful means of achieving personal goals. --Harvey Mackay

Visualization is a powerful tool you can use to help you focus more on life. It can be used to enhance a workout, improve focus in competition, help you relax, overcome an injury, and it can even pump you up. Visualization is a proven science and research studies have indicated it affects overall performance. Here are two studies to validate my point:

1) At Hunter College, 72 players from 8 college basketball teams participated in a study, whereby they worked on the mental aspect of shooting free throws. One group began each day's basketball practice with a relaxation technique, followed by visualization or mental rehearsal, in which they imagined every detail of their foul shooting. They pictured preparing for the shot at the free throw line, bouncing the ball a few times, raising their shooting arms with the ball balanced in their palms, bending at the knees, and releasing the ball toward the hoop.

Using this technique, the shooting accuracy of these athletes improved by 7 percent--a change so significant that coaches reported 8 additional wins during the season. These athletes were connected to sensors that measured their neuromuscular activity during mental training. The sensors showed that the same muscles used in Free-throw shooting was activated during the practice imagery.

Thus, on a subtle level, the body itself was going through the motions of free-throw shooting. Amazing!

2) Researchers at the Olympic Training Center in Colorado enlisted 30 college-age golfers, who were asked to work on their putting each day for a week. One group was instructed to visualize their sinking each putt, just before tapping the ball toward the hole. They were told to picture the entire process--from the backswing before the ball is struck, to the ball rolling into the center of the cup.

A second group was instructed to do the same, but with one change: in their imagination, they were asked to picture the ball veering to the left or the right just as it approached the hole, stopping just inches from the cup.

A third group practiced only putting, without doing any visualization. When the week was over, the golfers in the first group improved their putting accuracy by 30 percent; by comparison, the group who did no visualizing but physically practiced their putting showed improvements as well, by 11 percent.

Most intriguing, the middle group, those who pictured the golf ball straying off course, away from the cup experienced a worsening of their putting. Their accuracy declined by 21 percent throughout the week. They had pictured themselves putting poorly, and they did just that.

As you can see, visualization works. It is your highlight movie. It takes practice and consistency to implement it. Visualization begins with proper breathing. As a certified Performance Edge Coach, I learned this process through Doctor JoAnn Dahlkoetter, a sports psychologist consultant and author.

In particular, deep belly breathing is a great tool individual can use to gain clarity, get rid of clutter, and focus on the process. It is done by breathing in for 5 seconds, holding your breath for 2 seconds, and breathing out for 7 seconds. It is also important to push the stomach out as you breathe in and then bring the abdomen towards the spine as you breathe out. You do not want to put too much emphasis on having the chest rise. Deep belly breathing has many benefits from reducing stress, anxiety, lowering heart rate and blood pressure, and enhancing the bodies' organ systems.

Practice deep belly breathing. Take 3 deep breaths in and out and then write down how you feel.

Now that you get an idea of how to do deep belly breathing, the next step is to implement different elements. I am going to go through all the elements, and then I am going to have you create your visualization.

The first element is for you to pick a favorite place in nature (e.g., beach, mountains, and park) or an actual place (e.g., ball game, stadium, work environment). The reason behind choosing a place is to help you concentrate more on your breathing. Along with this element you want to include power words. These are words or affirmations you can implement to enhance your confidence. This is how it would work. I am going to use the beach as my example. Give it a try.

Before beginning, find a quiet place with no distractions. Close eyes and focus on yourself.

Take a deep breath in and as you breathe in imagine the waves of positive energy coming towards you, hold onto it and as you breathe out to let all negative thoughts wash away. Breathe in again and as the waves wash upon the shore gather emotions of happiness, calmness, and focus. Hold onto those emotions and as the water goes back into the ocean breathe out and let emotions of fear, nervousness, and clutter clear your mind.

One more time, breathe in and feel the big bright sunshine gleaming on your face and let this represent the success you are going to have today. Hold onto it and breathe out any doubts in your mind.

The next element or step in the visualization process is to recall a peak experience in your life. This can be a great workout, the competition you were in, or great work event. It can be something from your childhood. The only rule here is that it must be a positive peak experience. You want to do your best to focus your visualization on the positiveness. Let's do this one together. Use positive images and have the presence of mind.

Keeping your eyes closed...I want you to imagine a time where you had a peak experience. This could have been an event you excelled at, a day at work where you changed someone's life or memory of playing sports.

Now imagine you are actually at this event. Think about this day and who was with you. Think about how great you feel on this day before your event begins. You are rested, focused, and ready to go. During the event, you see people cheering and lots of smiles. You are feeling full of energy, motivated, empowered, confident, and elated.

You are approaching the finish line or the end of your event, and you can feel every inch of your mind, body, and soul fuel you through the end. Always remember that your mind-set is contagious and the positive energy you display moves you closer to your goals every day in life. Remember the thoughts, feelings, and actions you had before, during, and after this peak experience. Hold onto this image and visualize to energize...visualize to energize.

The last element or step in the visualization is to come out of the visualization. Here is how this step will work.

Now holding onto this image...feel yourself walking up stairs...and with each step you are becoming stronger and stronger. Step by step you are getting to where you need to be. Today is your day! Right now you are empowered to be your best! Get after it!

Now it's your turn to create your visualization. I will go over the steps again, then write out your own on the next page.

Step 1. Find a quiet location without distractions, close eyes, and focus on yourself. Think about a place in nature.

Step 2. Take 3 deep breaths. As you breathe in, think about positive thoughts, feelings, and actions. As you breathe out, let go of negative thoughts, feelings, and actions.

Step 3. Recall a peak experience or event (act as if you are there). Recall all physical senses and what happened that day. Who was with you? How did it make you feel before, during, and after?

Step 4. Come out of visualization. Use the staircase to imagine yourself stepping up and elevating your game.

Write out your visualization below:

Using Your Visualization

Congratulations on developing your visualization. Take what you wrote down and record your voice using your smart phone/tablet/computer. You can even add your favorite music in the background. Customize it however you would like.

After you record yourself, listen to your visualization regularly. (e.g., before you go to sleep, upon awakening, before a workout/ practice, or a competition/major event).

Use it to your advantage and remember you can change it at any time. You now know the process of how to do it. Enjoy visualizing!

Other Mental Training Techniques

Along with visualization, there are many different techniques you can use to train the mind. There are brain training games on the computer and even advanced technology services, apps, and programs.

Techniques that you can apply now can be as simple as creating your music play lists. For example, create some for keeping your mind calm and focused and then have some for getting you pumped up for your next workout/practice/event.

Use your phrases or acronyms. It can be as simple as the word focus. Write it out on a wrist band. Other examples are BM - Beast Mode and GRN - Get Ready Now, Stay Calm, Breathe, etc. Can even add a symbol such as a plus (+) sign.

Use imagery. Think about your favorite number, animal, or shape. Use the image to motivate you. For example, a lion can paint a picture of a heart and toughness in your mind. Another example can be to the number one that reminds you about being the best you can be daily.

Thought stoppage. Eliminate negative thoughts and replace them with positive ones. I had a professional foot volley player share this experience with me. He caught himself before a major tournament talking negatively about himself. To change his mindset, he looked himself in the mirror and began telling himself positive messages to get his head on straight. He went on to win the tournament.

Progressive Muscle Relaxation. This can be accomplished by tensing on muscle at a time. For example, during an event or game, you can squeeze hands together and then release tension. As you apply pressure use positive self-talk.

Concentration. In terms of concentration, it is important to focus on the things you can control and not the things you can't control.

Implement the 3 Power P's

The way we choose our words can have a big impact on the way we program our mind. "I want," "I wish," "maybe," "only if," "what if," and "I should have" are weak messages that you send to your brain. When you choose phrases like "I need to," "I am," and "I will accomplish this," then these are powerful words. I learned from my great mentor, Dr. JoAnn Dahlkoetter, author of Your Performing Edge, that the mind works with three Ps. She refers to these as her "Power P's." They are:

Power Words: Use power phrases to help you think into positive results. Phrases such as "I can" and "I will" are much more impactful than "I want" or "I will try." Instill power into your life by speaking with positive self-talk. Here are some examples of power words: energize, inspired, empowered, strong, focus, calm, excited, grateful, pumped up, ready to go, etc.

Positive Images: You are an artist in your own right. When you create an image of the life you want and hold onto that image, it will become real the more you see and believe in it! Paint the picture of the goals you have. Draw them, write them down, map them out, and act on them.

Presence of Mind: Have tunnel vision and focus on the things that you can control. What happens outside of your control should not be your main focus. Live in the moment, and put in your best effort at any given time, as this is your primary driving force. Focus on the things you do want, and keep your mind off the things you do not want.

Always assess your environment, analyze your next move(s), rehearse it in your mind, and then take action.

In all, these mind training techniques can be used to help you feed your potential. Use them to your liking and come up with your system for getting you to the next level.

Increasing your performance will give you:

- Higher self esteem
- More energy
- Improvement of mood
- A positive mindset
- A plan of action

The next section will go into setting your goals and creating a goal setting ladder for yourself.

Goal Setting

"A person should set his goals as early as he can and devote all his energy and talent to getting there. With enough effort, he may achieve it. Or he may find something that is even more rewarding. But in the end, no matter what the outcome, he will know he has been alive."--Walt Disney

Let's discuss goals. Outcome, process, and performance goals are great ways to measure your success. Understanding these goals will allow you to set sufficient goals to feed your potential.

Outcome Goals. These goals refer to goals that dictate the Outcome of an event. For example, your goals might be to win a race or be the fittest in the class. When it comes to the outcome, it is important to understand that you do not have direct control of the result. Focusing your expectations on just the outcome can lead to major disappointment. Setting goals that focus on the process allow you to improve every time you step onto the playing surface.

Process Goals. These goals represent what you can measure. Process goals consist of your physical (fitness/strength), technical (form/movement) and tactical goals (game strategy). When you focus on the process, it allows you to break down your performance and make adjustments necessary to improve. Some of the best athletes in the world are setting process goals regularly to feed their potential continually.

Performance Goals. These goals are about setting new personal records. As learned from the book: The Champion's Mind: How Great Athletes Think, Train, and Thrive by Jim Afremow, you can set goals that represent gold, silver, and bronze. For example, if you are running a 5k race your bronze time might be 24:00, silver might be 21:00, and your gold might be 18:00.

Along with understanding the difference between outcome, process, and performance goals; it is vital to make sure your goals are **SMARTER.**

S- SPECIFIC - Focused on the process.
M - MEASURABLE - Keep track of progress.
A - AMBITIOUS - Pushes you outside of your comfort zone.
R - RECORDED - Written down on a regular basis.
T - TIME PHASED - Set a completion date. (*Use Goals Card)
E - ENERGETIC - Keeps you motivated and energized.
R – REWARDING - Gift yourself soemthing and then set new goals.

Goal Setting Ladder

A goal setting ladder represents long term (yearly), medium (3-6 months), short (monthly/weekly), and micro (daily/weekly). I suggest developing goals for your personal life (e.g., Organize House), education (e.g., Complete Degree), and performance (e.g., Lose 15 pounds of fat, gain 5 pounds of muscle). I highly encourage you to write down your goals regularly. Remember that the mind can forget, but the pen does not.

Write in your goals below:

Long-Term Goals (1 year+)

Medium-Term Goals (3-6 Months)

Short-Term Goals (Monthly-90 Days)

Micro Goals (Weekly, Daily, Hourly)

Great job on completing your goal setting ladder. Demand perfection from yourself and do your best!

By writing down your goals, you give yourself a written agreement to stand by.

Goals give you meaning and they motivate you. Best of all they keep you focused.

Use this system for any major life goal you have and make it a fun process.

Share your goals with those close to you.

Let them know how meaningful they are to you.

After you accomplish them, go ahead and celebrate. You deserve it.

It's all about having a positive mental attitude.

Goals Card

The Goals Card is a wonderful tool to use to recall your goals and have it with you at all times. (Example card is below). Make a goals card (or cut out the one below), laminate it, and use it daily to infuse your main goals into your sub-conscious mind. The more you use it, the more you will think about it. Share your goals card with people who are close to you, and continually work toward it. Once you achieve your goals, make a new goals card and repeat.

My Goals

By: _____ I will have achieved the following:

_____

_____

_____

I commit to my goals. Signed _____

Attitude

"Weakness of attitude becomes weakness of character."
--Albert Einstein

Your attitude is a composite of your thoughts, feelings, and actions. The thoughts you choose generate your feelings, which produce actions. Your actions then produce the results you are getting in life. I like to use the PEP principle that I developed when thinking about attitude and how it relates to life.

PEP Principle. This means you need to have positive thoughts that can lead to energetic feelings, which will create proactive actions.

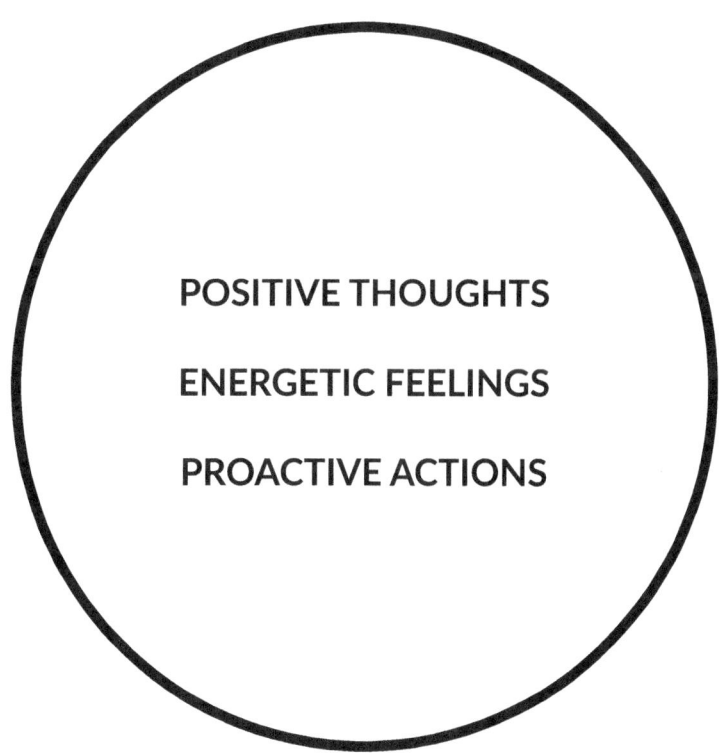

POSITIVE THOUGHTS

ENERGETIC FEELINGS

PROACTIVE ACTIONS

I have personally worked with athletes and individuals when they apply this principle; they get great results. This principle has allowed athletes to work harder on and off the playing surface daily. Use this principle and incorporate it into your life and see the positive changes happen for you. Go for it! It is important to understand the impact of the words inside the circle on the previous page. Inside of the circle represents responsibility. When you do not take responsibility for your thoughts, you start playing the blame game, and you step outside of the circle.

I believe we have all made mistakes in our lives; own up to it and accept the fact that you need to take responsibility for your goals. Those who play the blame game lose. If you allow others to make you sad or glad, this will weaken your potential.

Put your mind to work in your favor and optimize your attitude. Attitude has everything to do with the way you conduct yourself. When you have a plan for your performance, your attitude is easily elevated to the next level. Develop a burning desire to be great and do not look back.

I love the story of Ghandi when it comes to your habits in life. Ghandi was asked to help out a mother's child. The mother wanted Ghandi to have her son stop eating sugar. Ghandi responded by telling the mom to come back in a couple of weeks and he will be glad to help. Elated by his response, the mom could not wait to hear from Ghandi. After two weeks went by, the mom returned with her son, and the mom asked Ghandi to help again. Ghandi replied by saying, "stop eating sugar." The mother was shocked by the response and said, "that's it? Why couldn't you told him that two weeks ago?" Ghandi replied by saying, "because two weeks ago I was eating sugar."

The point of this story is that we must practice what we preach. When it comes to habits that we have in life, do not expect someone to change unless you are living that life yourself.

With that being said, let's evaluate your habits with another tool called success. I learned this concept from *Todd Durkin. The Success Training Blueprint: The 3 Essential Elements to a World-Class Business & Life.*

Purpose + Passion + Vision = Achieved Goals

Success Wheel:

Mark the number in the circle (on the next page) that relates to how satisfied you are with each category and then connect the marks. (1 - not satisfied and 5- very satisfied).

1. **Growth -** Rate how satisfied you are with the amount of time you invest in personal development, growth, and leaning from others.

2. **Financial -** Rate how satisfied you are with your financial life.

3. **Personal Life -** Rate how satisfied you are with your general health (e.g., fitness, conditioning, general wellbeing).

4. **Relationships -** Rate how satisfied you are with your family/ significant other/relationships.

5. **Performance -** Rate how satisfied you are with your performance. (Personal/Education/Career or Sport).

6. **Fun/Adventure -** Rate how satisfied you are with your free time, hobbies, and travel time. (e.g., vacations, arts/crafts, relaxation).

7. **Mind Training -** Rate how satisfied you are with your mental training (e.g., deep breathing, goal setting, and visualization).

8. **Personal Habits -** Rate how satisfied you are with your habits (e.g., cleanliness, organization, schedule, nutrition) in life.

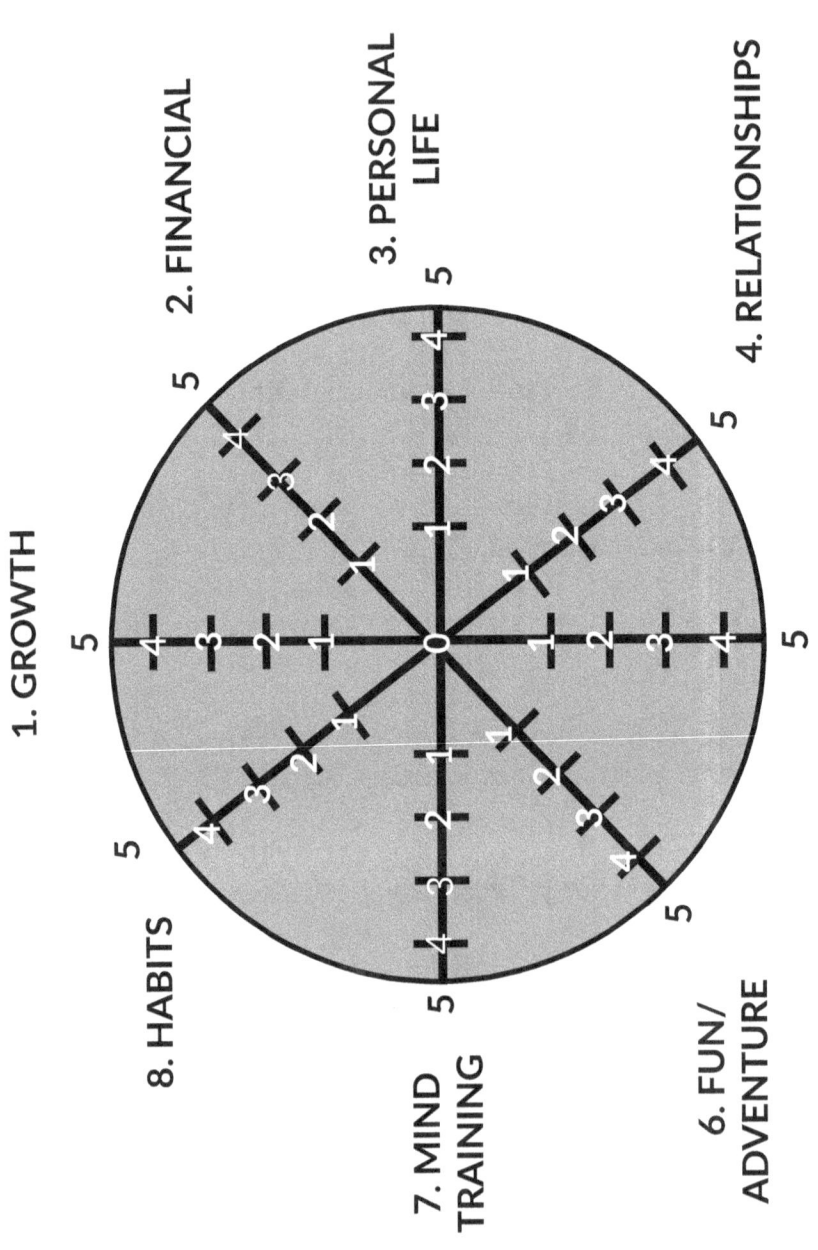

1. GROWTH

2. FINANCIAL

3. PERSONAL LIFE

4. RELATIONSHIPS

5. PERFORMANCE

6. FUN/ ADVENTURE

7. MIND TRAINING

8. HABITS

Now that you completed that exercise, connect all your dots so it makes a complete circle. How does your wheel look?

"Will you have a relatively easy time getting down the street with the wheel you have or are you looking at a very bumpy ride?"

Ask yourself, Where can I get better? Perhaps you need to **GROW** and begin to create change in order to get your wheel rolling down the street more smoothly. Let me explain.

GROW is an acronym that I came up with that stands for:

- **Get Your Mind Right -** purpose, vision, and goals.
- **Refocus Your Life -** assessments and goal writing.
- **Optimize Your Nutrition -** balanced eating habits.
- **Workout Smart -** weights, flexibility, funtional/sport specific, rest.

Focus on your peak performance with fitness, nutrition, and using a performance journal.

Peak Performance

"A man can be as great as he wants to be. If you believe in yourself and have the courage, the determination, the dedication, the competitive drive, and if you are willing to sacrifice the little things in life and pay the price for the things that are worthwhile, it can be done."--Vince Lombardi

We all seek to grow in life and be our best. I believe that we all have a tendency to fall into a comfort zone.

Peak Performance begins with your ABC's. This refers to Awareness, Breathing, and Concentration. Where do you need to bring more awareness to? Is it your physical game, nutrition game, and mind game?

Perhaps it's all three. What about taking time to breathe before you react to life. Before doing so, breathe and concentrate on what you want the result to be. For example, if you reach for an ice cream bar, how is that honestly going to make you feel after eating it? Again, be aware of what you are doing. Think before you react and focus on the results you want.

Where do you need to refocus your energy? How much time do you spend on working on your dreams versus entertainment? What's your vision? What values do you treasure in your life? Are you organized? Do you need to clean up better around your house, car, and school/workplace?

What technology can you use to enhance your current position? (Check out Udemy.com). What systems do you have in place? Who do you know in your industry or life that can mentor you and provide you with information to give you the extra edge?

If you are a student-athlete, who can you talk to, in other to learn what it takes to get to the next level? Find a way to connect with a professional athlete and listen to their advice. Plant the vision in your mind. Refocus your energy and get after it.

My purpose is to get you to think about what you are doing. How about your nutrition? Can you do better? Can you cut out more processed foods or supplements that are not the best for you. I highly recommend looking into products that are certified by NSF Sport and Informed Choice/Informed Sport if you play competitive sports.

Do your research and put the best quality foods and supplements into your body to perform at your best. Perhaps look into products that are gluten/hormone free, and organic.

"As far as nutrition goes, there are no secrets. Eat small whole based meals/snacks to support your bodies metabolism throughout the day. Drink lots of water and do it on a consistent basis."

The most important factor for athletes is to eat a well-balanced diet and to understand when to increase their intake of carbohydrates, protein, and fats along with caloric intake when needed. Also, it is important to monitor glycogen needs. As learned from the book, Physiology of Sport and Exercise, an athlete's nutrition plan should generally consist of 55-60 % carbohydrates, 35 % fats
(10 % saturated fats) and 10-15 % protein.

Every athlete is different and trying to figure out the exact ratio of carbohydrates, fats, and proteins and measuring them can be a pain to do. As a coach, I do not give specific dietary instructions.

For specific diets, I advise individuals to work with a registered dietician/coach specializing in sports nutrition.

Use tools such as Avatar Nutrition, My Fitness Pal, and other apps that you have discovered that work well for you.

The Way I see it: Realistic Nutrition Outlook

Maintenance Phase/Off-Season:
70% nutrition lifestyle/30 % eating in moderation/enjoying different **foods.**

Contest Preparation/Season:
80% nutrition lifestyle/20 % eating in moderation/enjoying different foods.

High-Level Competition:
90% nutrition lifestyle/10 % eating in moderation/enjoying different foods.

Types of Athletes:
- Endurance Athletes (e.g., cyclists, triathletes, runners, etc.)
- Endurance/Strength Athletes (e.g., soccer, baseball, basketball, fitness competitors, cross fitters, football players, MMA, etc.)
- Other Athletes (e.g., fitness enthusiasts, house mom's, everyday workers)

Take Action on your goals with the first step!

"The journey of a thousand miles begins with one step."
--Lao Tzu

In the book, *One Small Step Can Change Your Life: The Kaizen Way,* *author Robert Maurer* describes how taking the first step leads to change. There is a story of a lady who lacked the motivation to exercise. One day, a friend suggested walking in place on commercial breaks while watching television. As a result, this lady followed this rule, and it got her to ask questions and get moving to achieve her goals one step at a time.

You can apply the same strategy for achieving your peak performance.

Furthermore, it is important for the different types of athletes to learn what their body needs most.

Regardless of the type of athlete, I believe it is essential to eat foods that contain complex carbohydrates, essential fatty acids, and lean proteins. It is important to drink lots of water because our bodies are mainly composed of water.

Below is a list of quality foods/drinks/supplements that I have found to be very helpful in my quest. *This is just for information purposes only and not to be used to prescribe a diet or nutrition plan.

Lean Proteins:
- Lean tenderloin
- Chicken
- Turkey breast
- Wild fish
- Lean beef
- Egg whites
- Beans
- Lentils

Joint Health:
- Glucosamine & Chondroitin

Healthy Drinks:
- Almond milk (unsweetened vanilla)
- Coconut milk
- All natural/organic protein powder
- Kombucha (one with chia seeds)
- Coconut Water
- Vegetable juice/Vitamin C
- Black coffee/Green Tea
- Water
- 1 serving of alcohol

Starchy Carbohydrates:
- Mixed berries
- Green apples
- Bananas
- Mandarin oranges
- Whole grain wraps
- Ezekiel Bread
- Whole wheat waffles
- Brown Rice/Quinoa
- High antioxidant trail mix (raisins, pumpkin seeds, almonds, walnuts, goji, acai, & berries)
- Fast cooking steel cut oats
- Brown rice or quinoa pasta
- Brown rice cakes
- Whole wheat pasta

Fibrous Vegetables:
- Frozen vegetables
- Fresh Salsa
- Spinach, 50/50 Mix
- Green vegetables
- Kale
- Assorted spices for flavoring
- Green beans
- Asparagus
- Broccoli
- Cauliflower
- Peas
- Brussels Spouts
- Wheat Grass
- Spouts/Spirulina
- Kelp/Chlorella

Sweet Cravings:
- Dark Chocolate
- Agave Nectar

Fats:
- Assorted nuts and seeds
- Coconut oil
- Olive oil
- Flaxseed Oil
- Udo Erasmus Oil
- MCT Oil
- Ghee Butter

Spices:
- Himalayan Salt
- Black Pepper
- Curry Powder
- Nutmeg
- Cumin
- Tumeric
- Adobo
- Basil
- Paprika
- Garlic
- Ginger

Supplements:
- Vitamin A & D
- Emergen-C
- L-Glutamine
- Fish Oil
- Muli-Vitamin
- Echinacea
- Oil of Oregeno
- Elderberry Syrup
- Chaga Tea
- Manukha Honey
- Zinc
- L Carnitine
- CLA
- Ginkgo Biloba
- Coenzyme Q10

Portion Control

Weight Loss Plan		Weight Gain Plan

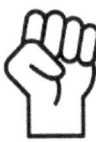 **Fist = Single Serving of Carbohydrates**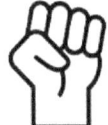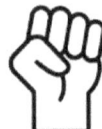

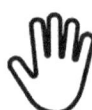 **Palm = Single Serving of Protein**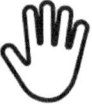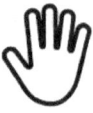

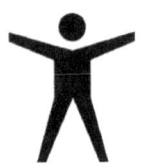 **Arms Open = Unlimited Serving of Vegetbales**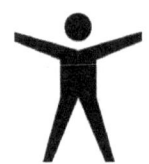

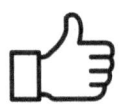 **Tip of Thumb = Serving of Healthy Fats**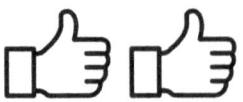

Example Meals

Example # 1

Breakfast – 2-4 egg whites and Ezekiel English muffin with 1 cup sautéed spinach
Snack – 2 Rice cakes with 1 tbsp. almond or peanut butter
Lunch – 4 - 6 oz. fish (tilapia, salmon, or mahi-mahi), 1 cup steamed veg's, and ½ cup quinoa
Snack – Protein Shake with water in shaker
Dinner – 4 - 6 oz. Chicken with 1/2 sweet potato and side garden salad w/ 1 tbsp. balsamic vinaigrette
Snack - Protein powder with water in a shaker

Example # 2

Breakfast – 1/2 cup Low sugar cereal with 1 cup unsweetened almond milk and 1/2 banana
Snack – Mozzarella Cheese stick, an apple or pear
Lunch – 4 – 6 oz. grass-fed beef, asparagus, and ½ cup basmati rice
Snack – Protein Shake with water in shaker
Dinner – Beef Stir Fri w/ mixed veg's and ½ cup brown rice
Snack - Protein powder with water in a shaker

Example # 3

Breakfast – 2-4 eggs w/ vegetables, ½ cup fruit or 1 banana
Snack – Small Bag of assorted nuts (10-20), Green Apple
Lunch – 2 - 4 oz. Boars head turkey and hummus in whole wheat or spinach wrap, tomato, spinach, and peppers
Snack – Yogurt, low sugar, natural
Dinner – 4 - 6 oz. Chicken with 1/2 sweet potato and side garden salad with 1 tbsp. balsamic vinaigrette
Snack - Protein powder with water in a shaker

* With Exercise, Recommended to take Amino Acids, Multi Vitamin, and Protein Powder of your choice
*Portion Controlled Meals are Key and to Eat Frequently Throughout the Day

Example Food Items

Breakfast Items:

- 1/2 cup- 1 cup Oatmeal with 1/4 cup of blueberries, 3-4 strawberries, and 2 spoons full of granola.
- Ezekiel English muffin with half banana and almond butter (try PB2).
- Protein shake: 1 scoop organic protein powder, half banana, 3-4 frozen strawberries 1/2 cup unsweetened almond milk, 4 ice cubes, (add water to make it less thick), 1 tbsp almond or peanut butter (use pb2 for less calories) or 2 tbsp of flaxseed or hemp seed, 1/4 cup oatmeal, blend together and enjoy.
- Organic whole wheat waffles - 1 to 2, apply thin spread of peanut or almond butter to waffles, add slices of banana or 3-4 strawberries on top.
- 3-4 Egg white omelet with mixed vegetables: made with tbsp of coconut oil or olive oil, and either 1/2 cup cooked oatmeal, 1-2 slices of Ezekiel bread, or whole wheat/Ezekiel English muffin.

Snacks:

- 10-20 unsalted mixed nuts
- 1/4 -1/2 cup organic granola
- Organic or greek yogurt
- Breakfast burrito made with 3-4 egg whites, mixed vegetables, and whole wheat wrap
- Protein shake made with water, protein powder, and 1/4 cup dry oatmeal
- Protein balls - 1/4 cup honey, 1 and 1/2 cup oatmeal (quick cooking, but DO NOT COOK) , 1/8 cup dark chocolate unsweetened morals, 2 scoops protein powder, 1/2 cup peanut or almond butter. *Consume 1-3 for a snack.
- Apple with 1 tbsp of almond butter
- Mixed fruit bowl - Blueberries, strawberries, acai berries, blackberries, apple slices, tangerine slices, etc.
- Organic rice cakes with hummus or almond or peanut butter (try PB2). Can also try cashew butter.

Lunch/Dinner:

- 4-6 oz organic chicken/fish/lean beef, with 1 cup cooked vegetables and 1/2-1 cup cooked quinoa, brown rice, or half-full sweet potato.
- Spaghetti and Turkey Meatballs – Make using a spaghetti squash and lean turkey meat.
- Vegetable Burger Sandwich – use 2 tbsp hummus or avocado, spinach, sliced tomato, spicy mustard and 1, thin bread sliders, and 1 vegetable burger.
- Stir Fry - prepare with mixed vegetables, olive oil, and your favorite meat. Stir in a big pot and enjoy.
- Healthy Meatloaf - made with mixed vegetables and lean ground turkey.
- Healthy Lasagna - made with whole wheat pasta, lean turkey breast, and healthy ingredients.
- Slow Cooked Chicken - place chicken in slow cooker. There are many recipes that can be used such as adding salsa, honey, curry, and many other spices.
- Breaded Chicken - prepare using organic bread crumbs or whole wheat flour. Fry in coconut or olive oil and enjoy.
- Brown Rice or Quinoa Bowl - make a rice bowl with sautéed vegetables, brown rice, guacamole, beans, and your lean protein of choice.
- Super Salad - add spinach, chicken, sweet potato pieces, olive oil and vinegar, mixed vegetables, chopped nuts, and enjoy.

Nutrition Chart

2 Week Example Plan

DAY 1	DAY 2	DAY 3	DAY 4	DAY 5
HIGH PROTEIN/ VEGETABLES/ LOW STARCHES	HIGH PROTEIN/ VEGETABLES/ MORE STARCHES	HIGH PROTEIN/ VEGETABLES/ LOW STARCHES	HIGH PROTEIN/ VEGETABLES/ MORE STARCHES	HIGH PROTEIN/ VEGETABLES/ LOW STARCHES
DAY 6	DAY 7	DAY 8	DAY 9	DAY 10
HIGH PROTEIN/ VEGETABLES/ MORE STARCHES	HIGH PROTEIN/ VEGETABLES/ LOW STARCHES	HIGH PROTEIN/ VEGETABLES/ MORE STARCHES	HIGH PROTEIN/ VEGETABLES/ LOW STARCHES	HIGH PROTEIN/ VEGETABLES/ MORE STARCHES
DAY 11	DAY 12	DAY 13	DAY 14	
HIGH PROTEIN/ VEGETABLES/ LOW STARCHES	HIGH PROTEIN/ VEGETABLES/ MORE STARCHES	HIGH PROTEIN/ VEGETABLES/ LOW STARCHES	HIGH PROTEIN/ VEGETABLES/ MORE STARCHES	

Fitness Program

I encourage you to workout smart. It is important to always do a proper warm up that gets your ankles, legs, hips, and upper body ready to do work.

When it comes to the main portion of your workout, look to do exercises that make sense for your sport. Each workout should target muscles that will enhance your game. I found that the following workout schedule works best for myself.

Push Day (Monday/Thursday) - workout chest, shoulders, triceps, inner thighs, hip flexors, gluteus maximus, and quadriceps.

Pull Day (Tuesday/Friday) - workout back, biceps, hamstrings, outer hips, small gluteus muscles, and calves.

Wednesday/Weekend - Functional Day/Rest Day/Sports.

Overall, choose exercises that focus on building your foundation. You must be able to control your body weight before adding another element.

In my experience, I have seen many individual's who cannot do a proper push up, pull up or squat that choose to add an exercise tool such as a balance tool, suspension trainer, or extra weight to the exercise. Please make sure you are smart with your workout and build your foundation. Make sure your workout program makes sense and allows you to progress properly. Consult with myself or the proper health care professional if you have questions about exercise programming (including off-season, pre-season, during season workouts, etc.).

When it comes to cardiovascular activities, it is key to understand the importance of doing intervals and recovery. Intervals are great because they challenge your cardiovascular system and cause your body to recover after completing a circuit. It trains your metabolism and makes your cardiovascular system stronger. A circuit can be done through metabolic workouts, running intervals, spinning, swimming, elliptical training, stair climbing, etc.

I recommend using a heart rate monitor to keep track of your target heart rate. Many heart rate monitors will calculate your heart zone based on age. Many heart rate monitors will calculate your heart zone based on age — research companies such as Polar, My Zone, and Garmin. You can even look into different smartphones. There are many other companies available. Do your research.

Stretching Program

Stretching is an extremely vital part of your program. A great way to evaluate your mobility, range of motion, and flexibility is to do an overhead body weight squat exercise.

Most people in their lower half have tight hamstrings, calves, hip flexors, and piriformis muscles. You might also have tight quadriceps muscles and weak inner thighs.

Upper body mobility is equally as important. Stretching the chest, lats, and shoulders will help in optimizing performance. If you have lower back pain, then work on strengthening the core muscles that support the low back. Work on all the components of your exercise and nutrition program.

Stretching helps complement and complete your wellness program. Clients I have worked with that take the time to stretch simply feel better.

To help support your program, you can do the following:

- Purchase a stretch band and follow the stretch chart to go with it
- Hire a stretch coach
- Join a stretching or yoga class
- Add 5-10 minutes of stretching to end of every workout
- Hire a professional trainer/coach/therapist to stretch you keep you accountable or set up a custom stretch program for you
- Stretch with friends/family
- Use the True Stretch Cage

Balance Program

Stability training helps strengthen ligaments and tendons in your feet and ankles. Exercises can consist of balance pads, stability balls, and single leg movements. Add balance exercises to your workout routine regularly. For example instead of doing a standing biceps curl with both legs on the ground, lift one leg off the ground and complete the exercise. You will notice that your left or right foot (whichever one is supporting you) is working more. In addition, you will become more aware of your core keeping you stabilized.

Increase your core strength, burn more calories, and strengthen your foundation by adding balance exercises to your program.

Example exercises:

- Body weight push up using BOSU Ball
- Body weight squat standing on balance pads
- Single leg bodyweight reach
- Single leg bodyweight squat
- Single leg stance doing a shoulder press or biceps curl
- Stability ball crunch or plank on ball

Functional Training

Add functional training exercises to your program to ignite your fitness. These exercises consist of anything where you work in multi-plane movements, bend, and rotate. Example exercises are:

- Diagonal Wood Chop
- Rotational Twist with Cable Cross
- Lunge with Rotation
- Lateral Lunge
- Ladder/Cone Drills/Box Jumps
- Squat press with rotation

Implement functional movements, along with balance exercises to mix up your workout routine and keep it fresh. View example workout sheet on the next page.

Workout Program Example

CARDIO	SETS	DURATION	COACHING TIP
Bike	1x/week	15-20 minutes	1:1 Ratio on Intervals
Treadmill	1x/week	15-20 minutes	1:1 Ratio on Intervals
Elliptical	1x/week	15-20 minutes	1:1 Ratio on Intervals

ACTIVE WARM UP	SETS	REPS	COACHING TIP
Body Weight Squats	2	15	Use Bar for Support
Band Reverse Flys	2	15	Use Green Light Band
Band Chest Flys	2	15	Use Light Green Band
Band Rotator Cuff	2	15	Use Green Band
Wood Chops	2	15	Use 6-8lb. Medicine Ball

ROUTINE # 1	SETS	REPS	COACHING TIP
Seated Chest Press	2	15	Seat on 4
Seated Row	2	15	Keep Shoulders Back, Core Tight
Leg Press	2	15	Seat on 5
Rope Pulls	2	15	
Ab Crunch	2	15	Leg Adjustment on 5
Weighted Ab Crunch	2	15	Keep Arms Straight, Squeeze Core

ROUTINE # 2	SETS	REPS	COACHING TIP
Seated Shoulder Press	2	15	Seat on 5
Lateral Pull-down	2	15	Keep Shoulders Back, Core Tight
Leg Extension	2	15	Seat on 4, Pad on Shins
Leg Curl	2	15	Seat on 4, Pad on 3
Low Back Extension	2	15	Leg Adjustment on 5
Weighted Ab Crunch	2	15	Keep Arms Straight, Squeeze Core
Bicep Curls	2	15	Bend Knees, keep Core Engaged
Triceps Curls	2	15	Pull down, come up to 90 Degrees

Stretches: Back, Chest, Hamstrings, Hip Flexors, and Shoulders

Performance Journal

A performance journal can aid you in becoming more aware of your thoughts, feelings, actions, nutrition choices, exercise habits, and performance. It can help you develop a system for improving your game and getting it to the next level. It will also allow the you to answer questions that occur during a competition or practice. For example, why do I say, "what an awful shot, I can't make those mistakes every time I lose a point." When Roger Banister broke the 4 minute mile in 1954, he constantly repeated messages to himself that he can do it. It was a mental breakthrough more than a physical. Within the next year, 37 runners broke the 4 minute mark. What a change in a person's belief system. A performance journal helps you to focus on yourself. Here are some tips for you below.

"Keeping track of your performance allows you to see your mistakes, make corrections, celebrate victories, and empower results!"

- Be here, now. Pick out and focus on the right performance cues to help you stay in the moment.
- Stop worrying about the outcome of the competition.
- Let go of what others might think about your performance; stop trying to read others' minds.
- Park distractions, from your life, that you might take into competition.
- Perform functionally; the opposite of trying to be perfect.
- Make it a goal to have fun, instead of being too serious.
- Narrow your focus on one simple objective when you perform.
- Keep it simple and avoid over thinking or analyzing what's happening. Stop judging how well you are doing on every play, shot, or routine; get to the next play, shot, or routine. Re-evaluate after the game (e.g., film study).

How to Use Performance Journal

Use your journal to keep track of your performances. It is important to keep track of them so you can review your results over time. I use this performance journal with my athletes regularly to help them improve in their sport. It's like keeping your grading system. It allows you to see where you can improve or continue to keep up the good work. For example, you might have a practice on Monday, and you rate yourself with a score of 6. The reason behind it can be a lack of energy. Your actions are to tweak your diet and make sure you go to bed early to get enough rest and be ready for Tuesday's practice. Another example can relate to a competition, and you give yourself a rating of 10. You played amazing and had the best result you could imagine. Your reasons why involve proper preparation and focusing on your game and not focusing on your opponent's game. Your actions are to celebrate by buying yourself a new outfit and resting.

Check out Hal Higdon for running programs or other apps/websites/ Programs to keep you on track.

Keep track of your workout/practice, cardiovascular activities, and nutrition. 7 days of example templates follow this chapter.

Day _____

Rate your practice/workout/competition (column 1), cardiovascular activities (column 2) and nutrition (column 3) on a scale from 0-10 (0-worst, 10-best) and describe why you gave yourself that rating. Lastly, describe what you need to do next time to make it better or maintain a positive result. *If no workout/practice/competition, please show in rating box. Describe as day off in rating and actions box.

ACTIVITY	PRACTICE	CARDIO	NUTRITION
RATING			
WHY?			
ACTIONS / GOALS			

Day _____

Rate your practice/workout/competition (column 1), cardiovascular activities (column 2) and nutrition (column 3) on a scale from 0-10 (0-worst, 10-best) and describe why you gave yourself that rating. Lastly, describe what you need to do next time to make it better or maintain a positive result. *If no workout/practice/competition, please show in rating box. Describe as day off in rating and actions box.

ACTIVITY	PRACTICE	CARDIO	NUTRITION
RATING			
WHY?			
ACTIONS / GOALS			

Day _____

Rate your practice/workout/competition (column 1), cardiovascular activities (column 2) and nutrition (column 3) on a scale from 0-10 (0-worst, 10-best) and describe why you gave yourself that rating. Lastly, describe what you need to do next time to make it better or maintain a positive result. *If no workout/practice/competition, please show in rating box. Describe as day off in rating and actions box.

ACTIVITY	PRACTICE	CARDIO	NUTRITION
RATING			
WHY?			
ACTIONS / GOALS			

Day _____

Rate your practice/workout/competition (column 1), cardiovascular activities (column 2) and nutrition (column 3) on a scale from 0-10 (0-worst, 10-best) and describe why you gave yourself that rating. Lastly, describe what you need to do next time to make it better or maintain a positive result. *If no workout/practice/competition, please show in rating box. Describe as day off in rating and actions box.

ACTIVITY	PRACTICE	CARDIO	NUTRITION
RATING			
WHY?			
ACTIONS / GOALS			

Day _____

Rate your practice/workout/competition (column 1), cardiovascular activities (column 2) and nutrition (column 3) on a scale from 0-10 (0-worst, 10-best) and describe why you gave yourself that rating. Lastly, describe what you need to do next time to make it better or maintain a positive result. *If no workout/practice/competition, please show in rating box. Describe as day off in rating and actions box.

ACTIVITY	PRACTICE	CARDIO	NUTRITION
RATING			
WHY?			
ACTIONS / GOALS			

Day _____

Rate your practice/workout/competition (column 1), cardiovascular activities (column 2) and nutrition (column 3) on a scale from 0-10 (0-worst, 10-best) and describe why you gave yourself that rating. Lastly, describe what you need to do next time to make it better or maintain a positive result. *If no workout/practice/competition, please show in rating box. Describe as day off in rating and actions box.

ACTIVITY	PRACTICE	CARDIO	NUTRITION
RATING			
WHY?			
ACTIONS / GOALS			

Day _____

Rate your practice/workout/competition (column 1), cardiovascular activities (column 2) and nutrition (column 3) on a scale from 0-10 (0-worst, 10-best) and describe why you gave yourself that rating. Lastly, describe what you need to do next time to make it better or maintain a positive result. *If no workout/practice/competition, please show in rating box. Describe as day off in rating and actions box.

ACTIVITY	PRACTICE	CARDIO	NUTRITION
RATING			
WHY?			
ACTIONS / GOALS			

As a refresher of this book and some additional tips, below are four things you can do to perform at your best.

1. Write down your goals daily. Focus on three things you can do every time you go to practice or work, and understand what you need to accomplish.

2. Get on a solid eating program. Plan your meals and workouts ahead of time. For example, on Sundays, plan meals for Monday through Wednesday, and then on Wednesdays, prepare your meals for Thursday through Saturday. Stay hydrated every hour. Use your imagination to discover what works best for you. Keep a journal of the foods you consume for the next few days.

Remember this: *"If you can't pick it out of the ground, fish it out of water, or spear it, then it probably is not the best food source for you."--Martin Rooney.*

3. Before you hit the gym, know exactly what muscle groups you are going to train, and design your program accordingly.

For Example:

- Monday--upper body or push workout
- Wednesday--lower body or pull workout
- Friday--upper body or push workout

The following week, switch your order. Weight training gives you cuts in your muscles and makes them toned. And do not forget to add functional, balance/core, and interval cross training cardio.

For Example:

- Monday--elliptical for 30 minutes on interval program
- Tuesday/Thursday--interval runs on the treadmill
- Wednesday--bike 30 minutes/yoga class
- Friday--stair climber 30 minutes
- Saturday--jog outside 2-5 miles
- Sunday - yoga or stretch class

Cardio will improve your energy, heart and lung strength. As an athlete, train for your sport. One day, train your linear speed (e.g. ladder drills, sprints, backwards runs, etc.), the next day go for plyometric training (e.g. bounds, jumps, box jumps, vertical jumps, quick feet, etc.) Then the next lateral speed (ladder drills, agility, side shuffle, lateral foot quickness drills, etc.). This will allow you to best prepare for the multiple movements that go on in your sport. Work at it on a consistent basis.

4. Give yourself an off day. I call this a cheat day! Go out, put your work away, go enjoy the fresh air, and socialize with some friends.

5. Consult with a fitness professional. Recommended to work with someone with a exercise science degree and/or national certifications:

- *NSCA (National Strength and Conditioning Association)*
- *ACSM (American College of Sports Medicine)*
- *NASM (National Academy of Sports Medicine)*

Look for the best certifications for proper screening and creating a specific plan for yourself. One of the best regional certifications is through *Dr. Anthony Abbott (Fitness Institute International)*.

Overcoming the 5 Fears of Performance

"Courage is resistance to fear, mastery of fear, not absence of fear."--Mark Twain

It certainly does take courage to overcome your fears and to lead the way. Trust me, it is much easier to follow behind others and go with what they tell you to do, or follow their lead. Whether this is relative to work or performance, courage is the seed you need to plant to overcome the opponent known as fear. We all have it, and there is no denying it. Fear can come in some forms but I want to focus specifically on the five fears of performance.

Fear of Change

"If there is no struggle, there is no progress."
--Frederick Douglass

The comfort zone is a term much used today to describe a mindset or state in which you feel safe. You feel great when you are in this condition. You are not too challenged. The comfort zone is a nice place to be. Ah, yes it is! If you feel satisfied with where you are, then do not change a thing.

Change is a difficult fear to overcome. Why? No one wants to be told what he or she is doing is wrong or that his or her way of training stinks. I have approached people and kindly questioned their training techniques.

The result is an instant defensive stance, and comments such as, "I have to do this because of my injury," or "Running hurts my knees," or "No way," or "I am too old to do what you do."

The truth is that change is uncomfortable. It takes courage to admit you are not getting the results you want, and admit you need to change your program. Change your results today by changing the way you think. Put your plan into action, do your homework, and the fear of change will disappear.

Fear of Losing

"I play to win, whether during practice or a real game. And I will not let anything get in the way of me and my competitive enthusiasm to win."--Michael Jordan

We all dislike it when we score poorly on a test or lose in a game. You have a competitive spirit about you. This spirit is what drives you forward and pushes you to want to be better. Fear of losing is inside everyone. Fear drives some people to be better, while it hinders others' performances.

To win in the game of life is to perform at your best every day. "Fear is false evidence appearing real." This means you create fright from the mind and transform it into something bigger.

Nervousness, getting the chills, is a good feeling before a test, event or game. This means you have done your homework and taken your activity seriously. But, fear will take over your mind when you shift your focus away from your game, and let obstacles or opponents (including yourself) get in the way.

Fear of Judgment

"Humility is nothing else but a right judgment of ourselves."
--William Law

The number one fear most people have is that of public speaking. We simply do not want to consider what others have to say about us. I have learned that no matter what you do in life, someone is going to talk about you negatively, and there is nothing you can do about it. Just accept that you are not perfect and will make mistakes. Get excited about messing up and people saying "No" to you. Let criticism fuel your goals.

You have to take an "I Can" approach, and move yourself to accept who you are as a person. Recognize the other side of you, the part that judges. You might like to dance madly, and yet not go out there and do it because you fear others' judging you.

Fear of Criticism

"You have to laugh, you have to be able to take criticism."
--Tina Yothers

Imagine you just walked into work or practice feeling great. All of a sudden your boss or coach tells you that you have been demoted or dropped down the line because you have been under performing. He or she says you need to be more specific with details on reports, or that you have been playing under par because you have poor technique. Immediately, you take it personally and may decide to complain to friends and family about what has just occurred. You never dig deeply enough to uncover the real truth, but allow your mind to tell you that you stink.

Fear, anger, jealousy and all the other demons haunt you. You are simply pissed off! You have reacted to the situation without asking specific questions as to what you can do to improve. You are afraid to speak up because you fear censure from your peers.

Self-examination is a good thing when you drop your ego and take responsibility for your faults. Criticism is what fuels the leader to be better. The goal of life is continuing to get better and focus on the things we can do right.

Fear of Injury

"A year ago I had a back injury and followed a good nutrition program to help speed up my recovery. I focused on exercise and staying healthy to get back out on the ice."
--Sasha Cohen

Injury can be fatal to many athletes and people. An injury can simply end your career in sports, or perhaps limit you with your workouts. The problem some people have is they take an injury to another level. I believe they can use it as an excuse and hinder own performance by conditioning the mind to believe something is wrong, when there is nothing of serious concern.

Check it out; if there are no major factors like broken bones, torn ligaments, or anything foremost that is standing in your way, then an injury can mean pain. If you hurt and complain about inconsequential pain, then you are setting yourself up for more injury. If you go into a workout or game thinking limitation, then your mind will create a constraint for you.

Feed Your Potential by putting together a plan of action that will help you either overcome a serious injury you have or help you conquer some hurt you have experienced. There is a big difference between hurt and pain. Sometimes you need to take a leap of faith and push your body to its maximum potential. Sometimes you have to take a step back to develop patience with your injury and then proceed through the steps to getting better.

Always, you need to condition the mind into thinking about superior health and strength. Talk to your body and move it in baby steps towards where you need to go. You know what works best.

Emotional Intelligence

There are four different areas to look at when examining emotional intelligence. The first two deal with being intelligent with the self and the second two deal with the social environment and relationships.

1. *Self-Awareness.* This is the ability to handle one's own emotions. It is important to become comfortable with the inside of who you are.
2. *Self-Management.* This is the ability to handle stress and communicate with others.
3. *Social Awareness.* This is the ability to handle social interaction.
4. *Relationship Management.* This is the ability to handle other emotions and conflict.

Let's discuss some strategies you can use to work with each area of emotional intelligence. It is important to note that information from this chapter has been learned through the book *Emotional Intelligence 2.0 by Jean Greaves and Travis Bradberry.*

Self-Awareness Strategies

Listen to your internal voice: Know what pushes your buttons and learn how to control your reaction by thinking first before you respond emotionally.

Do not beat yourself up: If you make a mistake, ask yourself instead, "What have I learned?" It's a learning experience; learn the lesson, correct the mistake and move forward positively. Write about the experience in a journal. Keep track of your emotions and what triggers them.

Self-Management Strategies

Fall in love with your emotional release habits: Music, singing, dancing, playing instruments, writing, reading, studying, working out and eating wisely are some examples. Perhaps even Yoga or Pilates.

Check yourself: Make sure you're expressing your thoughts when fully awake, rested and fueled with proper nutrition. If you feel deprived in any way, request to speak with someone about the situation at another time. Also, be receptive to what the other person's saying and feeling.

Social Awareness Strategies

Learn from others' mistakes and take note: You can write about it. You might come across a similar situation, and this will make you more aware of its pitfalls.

Greet people by name: People love to hear their names. Repeat their names numerous times to help you remember them. It shows that you care, and when you care about others more than yourself, you build trust with them. They are more likely to remember you.

Develop balance: John Wooden (famous basketball coach for UCLA) says it best: *"To have quickness under control, you have to be balanced, emotionally and mentally balanced. To have physical balance, you have to be mentallyy balanced...Balance is keeping matters in perspective, not letting yourself get too high, or not letting yourself get too low."*

Look people in the eye: Adjust posture and look people in the eye when you talk to them. It shows respect, focus, and builds trust.

Relationship Management Strategies

Give it your best: Always put out your best performance; this way you never question your effort. Remember the little things that pack a punch. Remember to use please, thank you.

Avoid giving mixed signals: We depend on stop lights to direct us. When they go out it creates chaos. Same for people we deal with in relationships. Match your words with body actions.

Be sensitive to others feelings: We all want to be heard. When someone shares information with you, listen and be there for them. Do not judge them and ask questions back to better understand their feelings.

When it comes to being intelligent with your emotions, use a journal to keep track of experiences and what caused you to react to people or situations. Write about how you can improve and develop your emotional control strategies to take your game to the next level.

*Social media is a great tool to use for sharing positive experiences.

Write in your emotional intelligent strategies below:

Mind Muscles

When it comes to using your mind muscles, you need to understand the importance of your lower level of thinking compared to the higher level. Individuals who have a plan for their lives and know their purpose, vision, and goals have an easier time coping with life. When you do not have a plan, your emotions can easily be persuaded up or down. For example, someone cuts you off while you are driving and you react. You might yell at them, give them the finger, or honk your horn. Yes, sometimes it may be a serious issue that could have caused an accident, but when it does not, do your actions have a purpose? Will the way you reacted lead you closer to your purpose, vision, and goals? If not, then do not act on your behavior. On the other hand, a higher level of thinking refers to using your intellectual mind. This is thinking with a higher purpose, and your higher level of thinking consists of six mind muscles.

"For thousands of years, scientists, theorists, and theologians have agreed that we all become what we think about."

So if we know this, then it is important to have a picture of the mind. There was a guy by the name of Thurman Fleet in the 1940s that created an image to represent how the mind works. Let's look at this image below.

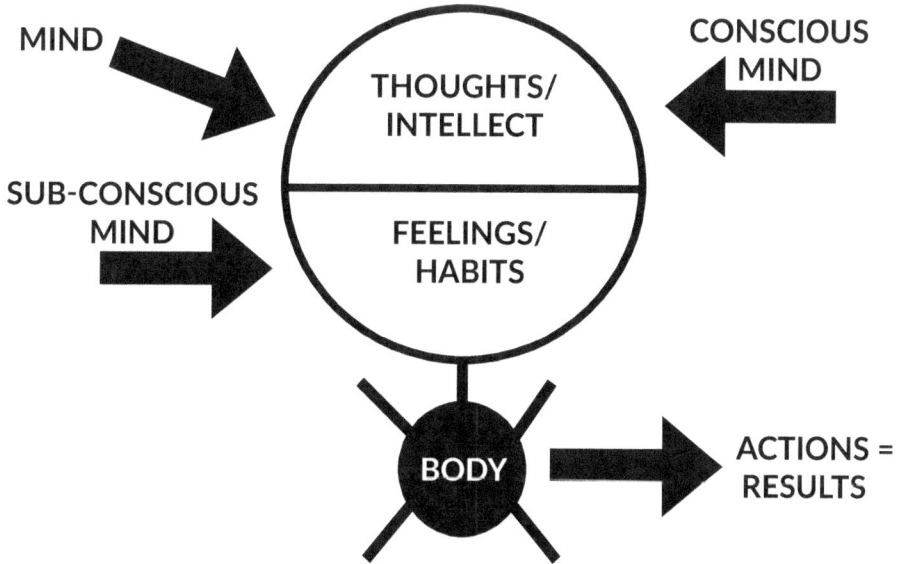

The stick figure is used to show that the mind is so much more powerful than the body. We choose our thoughts, our thoughts generate feelings, and those feelings create actions, which then produce results. The mind has two parts: the conscious mind and the subconscious mind. The conscious mind represents your thinking mind and the subconscious mind represents your habits, behaviors, and feelings.

This part of the mind does not think, it just does. Lastly, the body takes your thoughts and the feelings that are generated and creates actions. If you are not happy with those actions, then you have to change the way you think.

Understanding how the mind works relates to the six mind muscles. When you use your mind muscles together it creates a synergy that empowers you to fuel your soul and take control! On the next few pages, I will break down each mind muscle.

 # 1: Perception/How You See It. When you change the way you look at situations and use this mind muscle, your mind attracts the right things!

As human beings, we think in pictures, and when you have a clear picture of the way your mind works, then you will find more order and less confusion in your life.

As Wayne Dyer states, "Change the way you look at things, and the things you look at change."

Most of us gear our attention towards performing well on the physical level, without first seeking to create a plan for our minds. Take a step back and consider the way you see things. The way you think causes feelings, and those feelings get passed down to your body, and your body produces actions that lead to results. Positive or negative, you can choose to change your perception, and begin at once to take action toward your goals.

How do you see yourself--World-Class or Average? Is fuel left in the tank for you to drive further and work harder?

 # 2: Will/Focus. This muscle refers to your ability to focus on what's important. It is the focus, not knowledge or strength that will get you the results. Having laser focus will aid you with any goal you have in front of you.

The Power of focus can again be summed up by Vince Lombardi's statement: *"The difference between a successful person and others is not a lack of strength, not a lack of knowledge, but rather a lack of will."* I have met individuals who hold the highest degrees and certifications, have all the knowledge and potential skills in the world, yet lack one major quality; focus. This one important quality is the key to all success.

 # 3: Imagination/Creativity. This muscle is all about what is around us in our world. Take a look at the cell phone today. Remember when it was a block. Now, today it does everything. How about the way you imagine yourself to be? It is important to motivate yourself by focusing on the positive qualities you have and painting a picture of the life you want to create regularly.

As Napoleon Bonaparte stated, *"Imagination rules the world."* Along with the muscles of perception and will, imagination is of equal importance. You have a choice to imagine everything that can go right in your life, or you can imagine all the things that can go wrong. The mind is a powerful tool. You can think of all the wonderful things you want of your life, or you can imagine your inability to achieve them. As Jamie Paolinetti suggested, I repeat, *"Limitations live only in our minds. But if we use our imaginations, our possibilities become limitless."*

Use your imagination to think about all the things you do want. If you want to look better in a pair of jeans, or if you choose to increase your performance in running, then you need to partner your desire with the creativity of your mind.

Use your memory to picture all the positive experiences you have had and how you have overcome losses to achieve wins. We all have negative situations that set us back in our lives; however, you have the choice right now to take charge in favor of the life you seek.

A kid can play with a box and have more fun than using any other toy, because of his or her imagination. Fads and fashion start with imagination in mind. Use mind muscles to your advantage, and remember this, you have greatness inside you.

How do you want to use your imagination to move
toward your goals in life?

 # 4: Intuition/Little Voice. This muscle I refer to as the opponent. It is always on your case. Questions come into your head, *"should I eat the ice cream or not? Well, if I do I can get away with it."* You might tell yourself something such as you only live once. Use your intuition to stay true to you and empower yourself to focus on the things you want and not the things you do not want!

Ever question your talents and abilities? Ever battle with the little voice inside your head? The source of all our frustrations, successes and feelings about others begins with our intuition. This mind muscle determines whether you are drifting off course, or living purposefully--finding the answers and discovering whether or not the ideas that popped into your head can be utilized to your advantage. Will the thought in your head move you toward your purpose? If it will, then act on it the right way. If not, then write down the pros and cons of the idea, and justify your thought process.

Positive motivation from the experiences you have in life with its ups and downs is produced by the way you think. Your intuition permits you to know your inner truth. If you are unhappy with the thoughts and results you are getting, then you need to reprogram the mind through visualization, as I have mentioned, in terms of memory training. Two men who used their intuition to achieve their dreams and live their purpose when they were young were the Wright brothers.

After much trial and error, they finally made it happen in 1902. In 1903 they achieved the first powered airplane flight. They pitched their idea to the government, and it did not bite. Finally, in 1908, they demonstrated the airplane in action. Instantly, they became celebrities. The rest is history.

So what does your intuition tell you every day? Is it to begin your exercise program? Do you stop with the excuses, or are you programmed to reach for the ice cream after dinner? My intuition has driven me to write this program. I feel there is a huge need for training the mind into thinking clearly, and building an awareness of where you are now and where you want to go.

Remember to question yourself and continually repeat your purpose to yourself. Again THINK and ask the question: "Will this idea in my head move me toward my purpose? And if it does, then I am going for it!" Today is your day to act! Stop the excuses, procrastination, and simply act!

 # 5: Memory/Positive or Negative. It is important when using this muscle to remember all the success in your life. I have a saying, "celebrate life, and celebrate your victories!" These can be little accomplishments from losing a pound, having a healthy week of eating, or winning a contest.

As individuals, we do not take the time to stop and focus, to use our mental muscles to remember the simple things in life. We repeat things in our minds, like, "I am getting older." "I can't remember anything." "I have a bad memory." "I am bad with names."

We use memory in both negative and positive terms. Most of the time, we recall negative situations and do not give ourselves enough credit, or we use others' mistakes to make ourselves feel better.

Well, the truth is, we all have a phenomenal memory, and to train it, we need to be present and repeat names, saying them over and over again until they stick. Even using ridiculous association to help you works well. For example, "Jack on the attack," or "Anna Banana," or "Jill who likes to climb the hills."

 # 6: Reason/Ability to Think. You have the ability to think about your life and know where you are and what you want to do to get to the next level. Take the time in your day to think into the results you want in each area of your life. Be conscious of your thoughts and teach others to use these mind muscles to help them move in the direction of their dreams.

> *"Only one who devotes himself to a cause with his whole strength and soul can be a true master. For this reason mastery demands all of a person."--Albert Einstein*

As humans, we are unlike any other creatures on earth. We have an innate ability to think. The secret to life is we ultimately become what we think about all day long. Other creatures on earth do not have the ability to reason like we do, and know exactly where they are in space, or reason between what is right and wrong, as we can. Our minds are so powerful that we can instantly direct our attention toward a given object or task. We can also distract ourselves very easily and get off task. We have a choice whether we want to become rich and make a life for ourselves, or fall into a destructive pattern, and let the work be done for us, and just run through the motions.

Steve Jobs revolutionized the technology world. How about Mark Zuckerberg, who created Facebook? These two men have completely changed the way we communicate. Of course, there are other people like Bill Gates and many more people who have developed programs and technology for cell phones. The point is that they used their minds effectively, and they created both a dynasty and the future for our entire world.

I know for myself I can make plans, share events, and market and conduct business through social media and texting alone. You do not even have to pick up the phone and talk at times.

You have the time to think about your response, and to answer with adequate thought. Video games and internet websites, programming for the world, 3D printers, and many more innovations are coming to life. Our world is incredible. All these things come from the mind. Incredible!

We can express ourselves as never before. In my world, training and methods of enhancing performance have all been created through the making of new toys and the development of innovative techniques.

People that will support you, and people with impressive resumes who practice what they preach, are those you want in your sphere of influence. Think about the people you have in your life, and ask yourself, do they lift me and push me to be better, or push me down and make me weaker?

One of my clients was afraid to leave for college when it was time for him to go. He was scared because he was leaving his friends. I asked him this question: "Are your friends making you better?" With hesitation and a little awareness, he discovered that they were bringing him down. He changed his thought process and chose to surround himself with more leaders. Quickly, he became excited about moving closer to his purpose in life. Great story!

Write out how you can use each mind muscle to help you with your goals on the next page. Do you need to change your perception, add more focus, imagine the positive, fight off the opponent more, remember your successes, and think more about your choices?

Whatever the case may be, these six mind muscles are powerful tools you can use to fuel your soul and take control!

Use Affirmations

"Practice rather than preach. Make of your life an affirmation, defined by your ideas, not the negation of others. Dare to aim at the level of your capability then go beyond to a higher level."
--Alexander Haig

Affirmations are a great player to have on your team. Affirmations are short power phrases that you can use to elevate your success to the next level: phrases like "I am strong," "I am powerful," and "I am an athlete." At the beginning of this book, I spoke about how self-talk is a major factor in performance. It is important for you to understand that using affirmations will keep your mind on track. For example, you are invited to a party while training for a competition, and you feel you need to stay home to be focused. On the other hand, your head is playing games with you, telling you to have fun and worry about training later.

To help yourself out, use an affirmation like:

I am a strong athlete. I understand that discipline is needed for me to get to the next level. I will sacrifice for the attainment of my goals and put my desire to achieve my personal best in front of me. I know I have the focus to succeed. I surround myself with champions and seek the direction of doing my best. I am a winner!

Develop affirmations of your own, and use them along with your visualization, to empower you on your journey towards physical, mental, and emotional excellence. As I have said, my father used to sing to me at a young age, "This little boy will be a great man, this little boy will be a great man." I will never forget it! Thanks, Dad. Continually encourage yourself, and use affirmations with those close to you. You might be surprised at how much better a little comment like "You look amazing today!" will make you feel. Affirmations are great tools, and they get you involved in the game quickly.

Leadership

Leadership is a quality that gets developed over time. I truly believe that the best leaders in this world can lead themselves before leading others!

I take great pride in doing the right things in life and leading by example. As mentioned before with the story of Ghandi, it is vital to lead the way and not expect someone else to do it if you are not following your recommendations. There are exceptions to this rule, but for the most part, if you tell someone to eat healthier and then you are eating unhealthy, then come on Man!!!

Another part of being a great leader is having effective communication. (Read the next section on communication is king). A great way to talk to individuals is to use the Sandwich effect. This works by communicating with a positive talk followed by criticism and then finishing with a positive reminder. For example (using a soccer player) a coach can communicate to his player by saying, "You play the game well when it comes to passing the ball. Focus on kicking more with the side of your foot instead of the front. I am proud to have you on this team and appreciate your hard work."

Along with communicating effectively, it is crucial to coach individuals in an environment that is positive and allows them to grow. A task-oriented climate allows individuals to learn by focusing on characteristics that they can improve. This book, **Feed Your Potential**, represents a task-oriented climate because it is making you think about certain areas of your life (i.e., purpose, goals, habits, etc.). When you focus your game on the process of getting better versus an environment that is built on just winning at all costs (ego-oriented climate), then you are more eager to want to improve and be a part of something special.

I love to follow another acronym I developed known as the **3 Success S's – Strong Purpose – Secure Vision – Specific Goals.** As a leader, always seek out to have a strong purpose in life that gets you excited to get up every day. A vision that gives you hope and drives you to want to encourage others. Then, goals that make you feel fulfilled when you accomplish them.

Consistency is a major key to your success. Without it, you fall into the water and slowly drift away from shore. There are two opposing ways that you can be consistent. They are:

1. Having a consistent plan you never change, and getting the same old results.
2. Continual adaptation to change consistently.

I love the quote by Confucius, "When it is obvious that the goals cannot be reached, don't adjust the goals, adjust the action steps." How true this is, and yet, as humans we get into undermining habits that produce the same discouraging results.

You can be consistently negative or consistently positive. You know if you are that individual who has followed the same routine for years and even decades. If it isn't working, then change your darn routine, darn it! You want results? Then change the way you think. Develop consistency with the things you want, like leadership skills, and the habit of positive self-talk. Lose the negativity and boredom in your life. Do this by adding more color to your foods (add fruits and vegetables to your diet), changing your exercise routine, and thinking your way into positive results.

I have always been fascinated by how a spider finds its way and builds a web. Spider webs are incredible! Spider silk is about one-tenth the diameter of a human hair, but it has astonishing strength. It is ten times as strong as a steel strand of the same weight. The fascinating feature of a web is the spider designing it.

A spider possesses qualities of a leader, because, without any excuses, it uses its skill and thread to construct its artwork. If the web gets knocked down, the spider will just go back to work to design another one. Perhaps there is something in your life you want to act on, but are giving yourself excuses or conditioning your mind into believing you can't! What is holding you back from going after your goals? Immediately, you might be thinking of some reason why not. Time to think why I can! "Say no to weakness." Hold yourself to a higher standard. Expect more from yourself.

Communication is King

"Communication is a skill that you can learn. It's like riding a bicycle or typing. If you're willing to work at it, you can rapidly improve the quality of every part of your life."--Brian Tracy

We all have an audience that is waiting to hear us. They are waiting to receive our message and begin moving in the right direction. Whatever your passion is in life, it is important to live it. Far too many people just go through the motions and never attempt to realize their dreams because of fear, or difficulty communicating their message. If anyone understands, it's me.

Champions Communicate Effectively

Communication is the number one source of a team's success or failure. A true sign of leadership is effective communication. Poor communication can result in an interception in a football game, a poor pass in a basketball game, or a missed assignment at work.

The key to communication is to be positioned on the same page. For the members of a team, this arrangement often means getting used to one another. Your teammates need to trust you. It is the same in any relationship you have to learn about and understand each other, in order to be on the same page. You have to take responsibility.

Communication is easy when times are good; however, when matters take a turn for the worse, communication can go sour. Now, instead of playing a good game, you are in the battle of the blame game. The blame game does nothing to help you win; take ownership. If you are upset, calm your emotions and speak your truth to the person you want to express your emotions too. Be open and honest with the way you feel. When was the last time you needed to speak up but kept silent? The better the communication is between group members, the better the team will perform.

Use Music to Motivate You

If you are hoping to have a great workout, music with good flow will help you. For example, circuit training and cardiovascular training works best with rock, dance, and hip-hop music. Activities like mind-body classes and visualization work best with soothing, perhaps classical and light music. Which music better prepares you for your performance? I will give you a tip; as an athlete and competitor, the music that makes you feel calm and less anxious is advantageous. Do you need to make a change in the type of music you listen to? Use music to enhance your belief system.

> *"Whether you believe you can do a thing or not, you are right."*
> *--Henry Ford*

Believe in Yourself

Become the leader you are craving to be, and adopt this belief saying:

"I believe in my talents. I believe in the people around me. I believe that the purpose I have holds high meaning to me, and it drives me to be even better. I know that I might not be where I want to be today, but I am going to believe that I am who I want to be. I act as if I am already there, and believe that I own the goals I have set out to achieve. I am a world-class believer!"

Surround yourself with other leaders who support your dreams, people who understand what you are longing to do, and don't wish to persuade you to think another way. Those who believe in you are true mentors. Use their wisdom to motivate you to new heights.

I would strongly encourage you to do more research and study more about your area of expertise. Whether you are looking to grow in your career or sport, choose 5 books/programs you wish to study and write them down below. Be sure to share what you learn with others and get excited about leading the way! It's all about making yourself better and encouraging others to do the same!

1.

2.

3.

4.

5.

Growth

It is always important in life to have a desire to grow and become something more. Whether this deals with your personal, education, or performance; it is crucial not to allow yourself to become static. I always told myself as I got older, that my goal is to be in the best shape out of all my friends in each area of my game.

I always look at the positive in situations and if the situation attracts negativity, I do my best to find a solution and work with all individuals involved to make it right. I encourage you to avoid negative thoughts, jealousy, a weak mind-set, and excuses. Continually push yourself not to get comfortable and develop goals that will drive you to grow in each area of your life (mental, physical, emotional, and spiritual).

Here are some folks who have a growth mindset.

Wayne Gretzky has been quoted as saying, "It's kind of ironic when I broke in at 17, I was told I was too small, too slow and I wouldn't make the NHL." He's now recognized as one of the greatest hockey players ever.

Michael Jordan was cut from his high school basketball team. Michael Jordan said, *"I've failed over and over again in my life, and that is why I succeed."*

Anthony Robles won the 2010-11 NCAA individual wrestling championship in the 125-pound weight class, despite being born with only one leg. He finished his final year at thirty-six, and undefeated.

How about Einstein? His early teachers considered him an *"unteachable"* fool.

Over a hundred banks turned down Walt Disney before he got funding to develop Disneyland. He was also fired from his job at a newspaper for *"lacking ideas."* He also experienced several bankruptcies before he was able to develop Disneyland.

Thomas Edison is known as one of the most prolific inventors in history. When Thomas was four, he was sent home from school with a note. The note told his mother that she was to remove her son from school because he was *"too stupid to learn."* Thomas' mother decided to teach him herself. He had only three months of formal schooling, yet went on to create numerous inventions, such as the phonograph.

Henry Ford, Bethany Hamilton (Soul Surfer), Dara Torres (Olympic Swimmer), and Kyle Maynard (a wrestler who was born with a congenital amputation to the forearms and lower legs), are among many other leaders who have a strong growth mindset.

I will conclude with this story:

An ancient Indian sage was teaching his disciples the art of archery. He put up a wooden bird as the target, and asked them to aim at the eye of the bird. The first disciple was asked to describe what he saw. He said, "I see the trees, the branches, the leaves, the sky, the bird and its eye." The sage asked this disciple to wait. Then he asked the second disciple the same question, and he replied, "I only see the eye of the bird." The sage said, "Very good, then shoot." The arrow went straight, and hit the eye of the bird.

What is the moral of the story? Unless we focus, we cannot achieve our goal. It is hard to focus and concentrate, but it is a skill that can be learned. Develop *"tunnel vision"* in your game. Focus on what you can do best, and do not allow others or yourself to interfere with your concentration. Be your champion.

Continue to grow. Use the skills learned in this book to fuel your soul and take control!

What can you do to continue to grow and **Feed Your Potential**?